Flora's Fragrances

Essential Oil Blends to Enhance your Spiritual Practice & Life

"I am always captivated by Flora's work, from her amazing videos to her wonderful blog, so when she invited me to lend an "aromatic" hand in this book, I was thrilled! Her love for essential oils, and her innate understanding of the natural world comes through on every page. Flora has created a book that is a must-have for either the magical cabinet or the essential oil enthusiast looking beyond conventional aromatherapy. I will surely keep a copy in my school library!

~ **Liz Fulcher**, Owner of AromaticWisdomInstitute.com

"Flora's book is practical, down-to-earth, and filled with easy to follow recipes that are sure to enhance your Spiritual Practice."

~ **Sunny Dawn Johnston**, Author of Invoking the Archangels

"Flora has lovingly infused her essence and high-vibration into her book, **Flora's Fragrances: Essential Oil Blends to Enhance your Spiritual Practice & Life**. Sharing her personal private collection of recipes, she offers you detailed information to ensure a positive experience as you awaken and enhance your own spiritual practice with essential oil blends. As an Intuitive Medium, Reiki Master, and Spiritual Teacher, I highly recommend that you include this book in your spiritual tool box."

~ **Shelly Wilson** http://shellyrwilson.com

"Well she's done it again! **Flora's Fragrances - Essential Oil Blends to Enhance Your Spiritual Practice & Life**" is a fun, real life approach to aromatherapy for the spiritual practitioner. In each chapter Flora shares her knowledge and provides the reader with easy to follow recipes for essential oil blends that can do everything from lift your spirits to soothe your soul. Everyone from the first timer to the seasoned Aroma Therapist will find this guide a valuable addition to their resource collection."

~ **Rai Smith**, Elemental Allure

"Flora Peterson has succeeded once again in providing us a power-packed book of motivational inspiration. **Flora's Fragrances** is a welcomed addition to any aromatherapist's bookshelf, whether you're a newbie or an experienced pro. Unlike many how-to books, this one is super-practical and gets right to the point. Flora delivers essential oil blends for just about anything you can dream up. This book is short on the fluff and fillers, yet packed with useful multipurpose recipes. This book is one that I'll be referring to often while also recommending to my students, especially since Flora incorporates the vibrational frequencies of crystals in some of her recipes to enhance her oil blends.

Whether you'd like to balance your chakras, heal a headache, celebrate a time of the year or simply relax, you'll discover versatile aromatherapy inspiration galore within the following pages."

~ **Hibiscus Moon**, Founder of the Hibiscus Moon Crystal Academy, Author of *Crystal Grids: How and Why They Work*

"Flora brings two powerful alternative therapies (crystal healing and aromatherapy) together for a fun and refreshing look at creating your own scents and fragrances that will not only leave you feeling inspired, but refreshingly energized in mind, body and spirit."

~ **Dr. Veronica "Nika" Dearing,** Holistic Health and Wellness Specialist

---

"What I love about Flora's books is she always keeps them simple without sacrificing the most important information. Her past books and video's always seem to give me whatever information I'm am looking for and can't seem to find any place else. She does this once again with her newest publication **Flora's Fragrances.**"

~ **Donna Virgilio,** Psychic Advisor, 12Radio Host and Author of Goddess Horoscopes at 12listen.com. Donna also leads Goddess Tours around the world. **www.donnavirgilio.com**

Flora's Fragrances

Essential Oil Blends To Enhance Your Spiritual Practice & Life

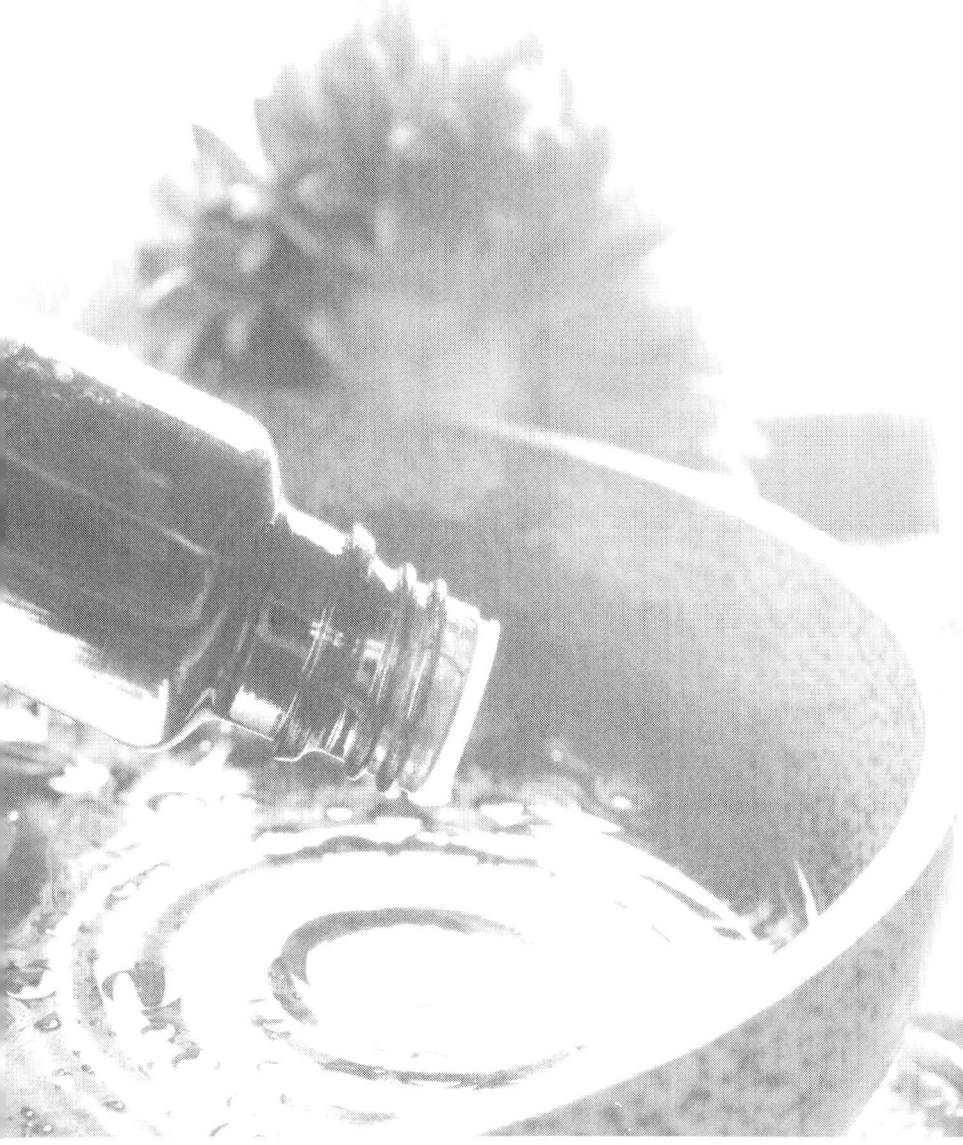

Flora's Fragrances

Essential Oil Blends To Enhance Your Spiritual Practice & Life

Maria,

Thank you for all your support over the years. It truly means SO much to me. Lots of Light.

Flora

By Flora Peterson

Flora's Fragrances ~ Essential Oil Blends To Enhance Your Spiritual Practice & Life
Copyright © 2013 by Flora Peterson and FloraSage Therapies LLC

No portion of this publication may be reproduced or transmitted in any form or by any means electronic or mechanical, including but not limited to, photocopying, recording or by any information storage and retrieval system, without the prior written permission of the publisher and author. Reviews may quote brief passages for educational purposes only.

First Edition, 2013

Published by Flora Peterson and FloraSage Therapies LLC
Photo credits:
Cover: Image ID: 59753101 Copyright: Subbotina Anna ~ ShutterStock.com
Section Pages: Image ID: 74566300 Copyright: Sergey Mironov ~ ShutterStock.com
Photo of Flora: Photography Mike's Digital Images
Hair: Shelli Jent ~ Style by Shelli
[https://www.facebook.com/pages/Style-by-Shelli/149361808429166]

All Recipes © FloraSage Therapies LLC

ISBN-13: 978-1481054614
ISBN-10: 1481054619

All Rights Reserved

The material in this book is not meant to treat any medical condition as diagnosed by any qualified medical practitioner. Since the use of essentials by others is beyond the author's and publisher's control, no expressed or implied guarantee as to the effects of their use can be given nor liability taken. Any application of the recommendations set forth in the following pages is at the reader's sole risk. Essential oils are to be used at the readers own discretion. The author and publisher disclaim any liability arising directly or indirectly from the use of this book and assume no responsibility for any actions taken.

~ SPECIAL NOTE OF THANKS ~

I'd like to thank Liz Fulcher, Owner of the fabulous AromaticWisdomInstitute.com, for lending her professional expertise, knowledge and wisdom to not only me but to you as the reader. Her corrections, recommendations and Latin binomials are sprinkled throughout this book and because of them the book you hold in your hand is of the highest standards. In the event where she has added a paragraph or sentence it will appear in the text in *italics*.

Thank you Liz!

"Living is about capturing the essence of things. I go through my life every day with a vial, a vial wherein can be found precious essential oils of every kind! The priceless, fragrant oils that are the essence of my experiences, my thoughts. I walk inside a different realm from everybody else, in that I am existing in the essence of things; every time there is reason to smile, I hold out my glass vial and capture that drop of oil, that essence, and then I smile. And that is why I have smiled, and so you and I may be smiling at the same time but I am smiling because of that one drop of cherished, treasured oil that I have extracted. When I write, I find no need to memorize an idea, a plot, a sequence of things: no. I must only capture the essence of a feeling or a thought and once I have inhaled that aroma, I know that I have what I need."

— C. JoyBell C.

Aromatherapy and Essential Oil blends create the opportunity for you to create an environment that helps to influence the way you think and feel. Using them, not only in your everyday life but your Spiritual practice can give you a sense of peace, harmony, balance and confidence in your practice and life.

Table of Contents

Welcome	21
This & That	23
Warnings, Precautions & Disclaimers	31
Spray Blends	37
Everyday Oil Blends	43
Massage Blends	51
Chakra Oils	57
Solar Cycle Blends	65
Lunar Cycle Blends	71
Lotion Blends	77
How to Create Your Own Blends	83
Essential Oil Attributes	89
Essential Oil Worksheet Pages	95
Recommended Suppliers	121
References & Recommended Reading	127
The Next Step	133
About Flora	137
Write To the Author	139
Connect with Flora online	141

Hello There & Welcome!

I am so excited that you decided to enter the world of Essential oils and blends. Yay!

Loving perfumes and scented lotions my whole life, I was somewhat distraught when after having my second child I became very sensitive to fragrance oils (aka, synthetic oils, fragrance oils and most manufactured scents). So, I began to experiment and blend my own scents for Spiritual and everyday use, using Essential Oils. As an avid hobbyist of this craft I would frequently create blends for my friends and family.

In 2010 I began selling a few of my oil blends in my online store and was delighted at the positive feedback about them. Having moved to an inventory-free store, since then, I have been inundated with requests for my oil blends. The birth of this book is a result of those requests.

So I decided to share my recipes with YOU! Yay!!!

In this book you will find all the Essential Oil recipes from my personal private collection of recipes I have crafted over the years that I find myself turning to time and time again. I hope you enjoy these recipes as much as I do! Yay!!!

Flora Peterson

This & That

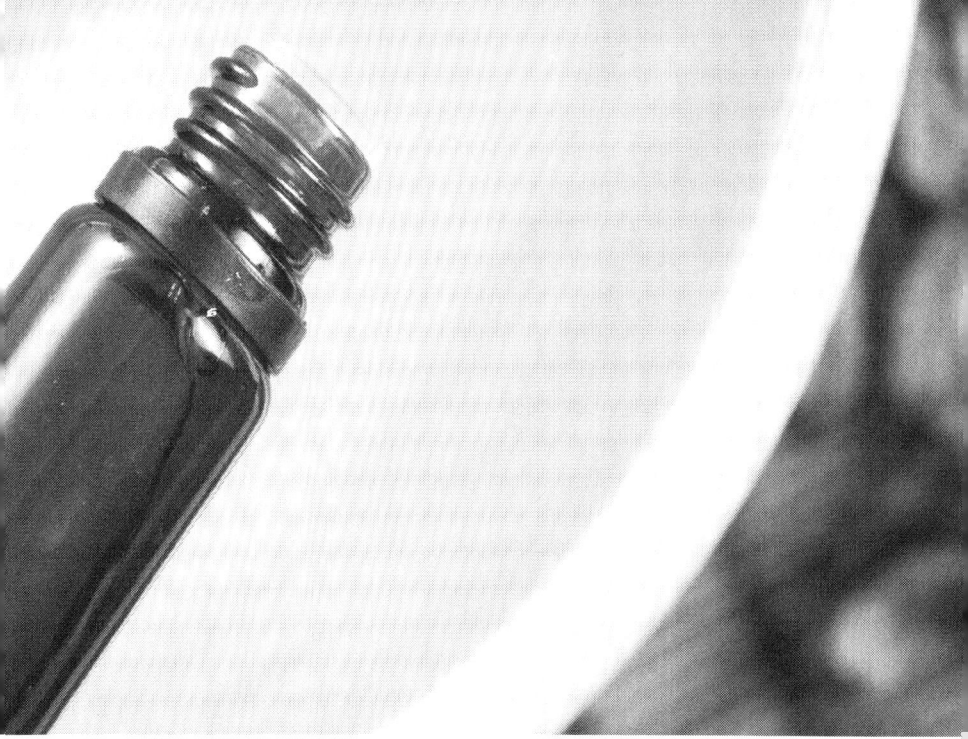

How to use this book

I am an avid hobbyist when it comes to Essential Oils and blending them. I am not a Certified Aromatherapist and have no formal training in this art. I have done extensive research on Essential Oils for my own personal practice and use them to enhance my Spiritual practice and life. Many if not all of my blends have been channeled for a specific use in my practice.

As you are reading the blends, I recommend you use your Higher Self, (ie..Intuition, Inner Knowing, etc..) to see if a blend is right for you and your practice.

There are worlds of possibilities when it comes to blending and creating with oils. I hope you have as much fun crafting with them as I do.

Preparing to create your blends

To prepare for creating blends I recommend the following:
1. Read the recipe through first
2. Be sure you are not sensitive, allergic etc to any Essential Oils used in the blend
3. Gather all items needed for blend
    a. Essential Oil, Absolute, CO2
    b. Base Oil
    c. Distilled or Spring water
    d. Crystal (if called for in recipe)
    e. Herb, root or other items (if called for in recipe)
    f. Label for bottle
    g. Unscented Lotion (if creating a lotion)
    h. Vessel for your blends
    i. Grapefruit Seed Extract to preserve your blends

4. Boil your vessel items (ie, spray bottle, dropper bottle, spray top, dropper top, etc...) to ensure they are properly sterilized before creating your blend. This will ensure no bacteria or other "what-not's" are in your blend.
5. Wash your hands and the surface you will be preparing your blend on thoroughly.
6. Create your blend
7. Enjoy!

I recommend you blend oils with a carrier or water before using on skin. Using oils "neat" (undiluted) could be harmful to your skin or body.

Always test oils to see if your skin may be sensitive to that particular oil before using it in a blend.

Always take the highest precautions while blending oils to be sure the oil does not come in contact with your skin while mixing. [Please see the next section on Warnings, Precautions and Disclaimers for more safety information.]

Essential Oils, Absolutes and CO2's

All recipes I featured in this book use pure Essential Oils, Absolutes or CO2s. I cannot guarantee your success if using "fragrance oils" as they are synthetically created and the quality varies based on manufacturer.

To ensure your blend will last a long time I recommend you purchase high quality, organic, pure Essential Oils. After each Essential Oil in the recipes I will put EO that will signify Essential Oil. For an Absolute and CO2 I will indicate as such.

Other Ingredients

Many of my oil blends contain crystals, to include Citrine chips; I use the power of Citrine as a natural way to keep my oil blends energetically fresh.

I also use dried herbs, seeds, spices or things found in nature. I feel that these ingredients add complexity and depth to the blend like nothing else can.

Spray Blends

All spray blend recipes are for a 1 oz spray bottle. I recommend you put in the ingredients as they are listed in the recipe and then fill the bottle to the shoulder with distilled or spring water.

Oil Blends

All oil blend recipes are for a 15 ml dropper bottle with a dropper insert so you can count out your drops. *(Avoid tops with rubber dropper bulbs as the oils will destroy the rubber.)* I recommend you put in the ingredients as they are listed in the recipe and then fill the bottle to the shoulder with a carrier oil of your choosing.

Massage Blends

All massage blends are added to a larger bottle of base or carrier oil. The recipes in this book are for a 2 oz bottle of carrier oil plus Essential Oil(s). Grape Seed, Avocado and Jojoba are wonderful massage oils.

LOTION BLENDS

All lotion blends are added to a base of any unscented lotion that you have available. See resources for a list of recommended lotions. The recipes in this book are for a 4 oz jar filled with unscented lotion plus Essential Oil(s). There are many unscented lotion brands to choose from; I recommend you purchase a high quality lotion for the blends you make.

CARRIER OR BASE OILS

Each carrier or base has a varying shelf life. I recommend you create small batches with fresh oils that have a shelf life comparable to your blend. [ie…for a blend you will use quickly, you can choose the base accordingly.] For the oil blends I recommend you use one or more of the following oils as a nice base for your essential oils:

- Jojoba (Longest shelf life of them all) ~ 10+ years
- Avocado ~ 1 – 2 years
- Sweet Almond ~ 1 year
- Apricot ~ 6 – 9 months
- Grape seed ~ 3 – 6 months

PRESERVING YOUR BLENDS

For blends you may not use up within six months, I recommend you purchase some liquid "Grapefruit Seed Extract" also called GSE. You can get this at most natural food stores or online. Place one drop of GSE in each blend before sealing and gently tip to blend the GSE with the mixture.

STORING YOUR BLENDS

Be sure to store your blends in a dark, cool place to ensure the Essential Oils will not deteriorate. *If they are exposed to direct sunlight, heat or oxygen, the essential oils may break down (a process called oxidation). Oxidized Essential Oils can be potential skin irritants and sensitizers.*

LABELING YOUR BLENDS

Be sure to label and date your blends when you make them so you know; what blend it is, when you made it and how long it will be good for.

VARIOUS OTHER METHODS TO USE ESSENTIAL OILS

There are many different ways to use Essential Oils that I do not explore in this book. Other methods are:

- In the Bath
- On Clothing
- As a Compress
- On a Cotton Swab
- In a Diffuser
- In a Dressing
- In a Face Mask
- In Face Oil
- As a Face Tonic
- In a Foot Bath
- As a Friction – Rubbing method created using EO and rubbing alcohol
- While Gardening
- As a Gargle
- On a Gauze
- As a High Dilution
- In a Hot Tub
- In a Humidifier
- In a Steam Inhalation Device or bowl of hot water
- In a Medicine
- As a Mouthwash
- Neat – (undiluted)

- As a Scalp Treatment
- In Shampoos
- In a Shower
- On Flowers
- On a Tissue
- As a Wash

If you would like more information on how to work with Essential Oils using the methods listed, please refer to the Recommended Reading list in the back of the book.

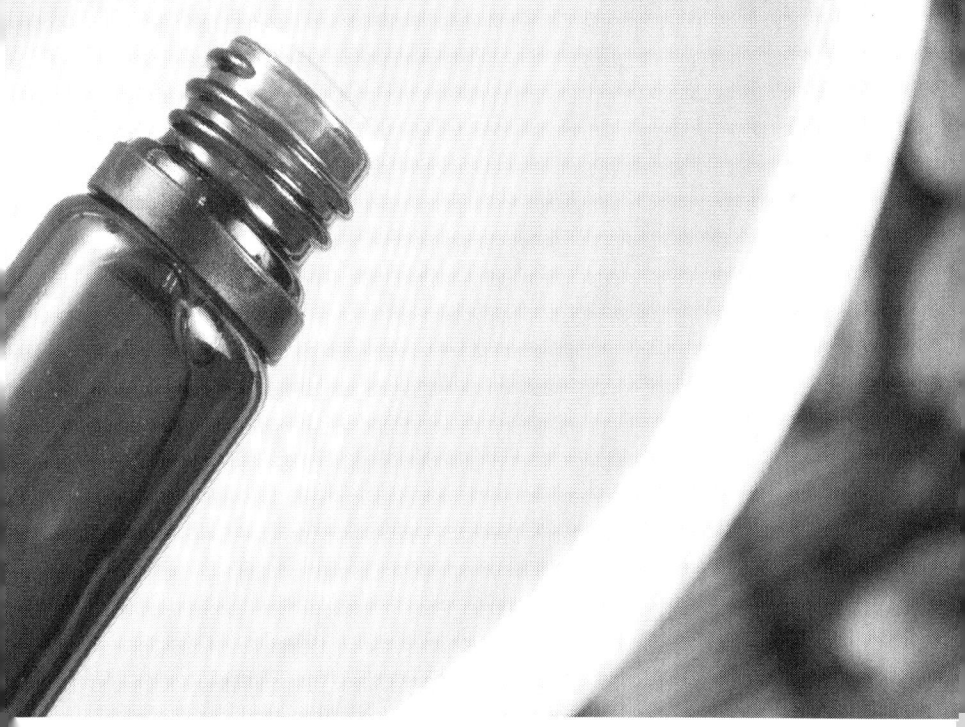

Warnings Precautions & Disclaimers

Disclaimer

I am an avid hobbyist when it comes to Essential Oils and blending them. I am not a Certified Aromatherapist and have no formal training in this art. I do not claim to know it all about Essential Oils and their uses. I recommend consulting a Certified Aromatherapist before you use any Essential Oil or creating any blends you plan to place on your body.

I have included a number of resources in the back of this book for further reading, which I have found to be invaluable in my personal study and growth as a hobbyist. I especially love *Advanced Aromatherapy: The Science of Essential Oil Therapy*, by Kurt Schnaublt. In this book the author discusses in detail how each Essential Oil: enters the body, how it is metabolized in the body, which organ the Essential Oil passes through, and how it is expelled from the body. Some Essential Oils come out via the breath, feces, sweat; it is all quite fascinating to say the least.

This is why it is so imperative for those with medical conditions seek the advice of a trained professional before using and Essential Oils due to the influences they can have on certain organs or systems.

Warnings & Precautions

Do not use these oils as they are considered unsafe:

- Ajowan
- Almond Bitter
- Buchu
- Bolo Leaf
- Calamus
- Camphor
- Cassia
- Costus
- Horseradish
- Mugwort
- Mustard
- Parsley Seed
- Pennyroyal
- Rue
- Sassafras
- Savin
- Tansy
- Thuja
- Wintergreen
- Wormseed
- Wormwood

Do not use these oils during pregnancy:
(or consult a professionally Qualified Aromatherapist)

- Angelica
- Basil
- Birch
- Bay
- Cedarwood
- Chamomile
- Caraway
- Clary Sage
- Carrot Seed
- Cinnamon
- Cumin
- Cypress
- Fennel
- Calbanum
- Hops
- Hyssop
- Jasmine
- Juniper
- Mace
- Marjoram
- Myrrh
- Nutmeg

- Organium
- Parsley
- Peppermint
- Rose
- Rosemary
- Sage
- Santolina
- Savory
- Tarragon
- Thyme (*Thymus vulgaris*)
- Valerian
- Wintergreen

Do not use these oils if you experience epilepsy:

- Fennel
- Hyssop
- Sage
- Wormwood
- Rosemary
- Peppermint
- Spike Lavender

If you have any of the following Special Considerations Please Do Not Use Essential Oils unless Cleared by Your Physician:

- Alcoholism
- Substance Addiction
- Pre & Post-Operative
- Are Pregnant
- Chronic Pain
- Terminal Illness
- On Medication
- Radiation Therapy
- Child under 12 years of age

If you have Sensitive Skin Please Avoid Using:

- Basil
- Bay
- Birch
- Black Pepper
- Cinnamon
- Clove
- Cumin
- Fennel

- Fir
- Ginger
- Lemon
- Lemongrass
- Lemon Verbena
- Oregano
- Parsley Seed
- Peppermint
- Pimento Berry
- Pine
- Thyme – ct thymol
- Wintergreen

Essential Oils NOT To Be Used on Skin Before Exposure to Sunlight:

- Angelica
- Bergamot
- Cumin
- Grapefruit
- Lemon
- Lemon Verbena
- Lime
- Yuzu
- Tangerine
- Manderine

Source: Schnaublet 1998 & Worwood 2003

Please use the following blends in this book at your own risk.

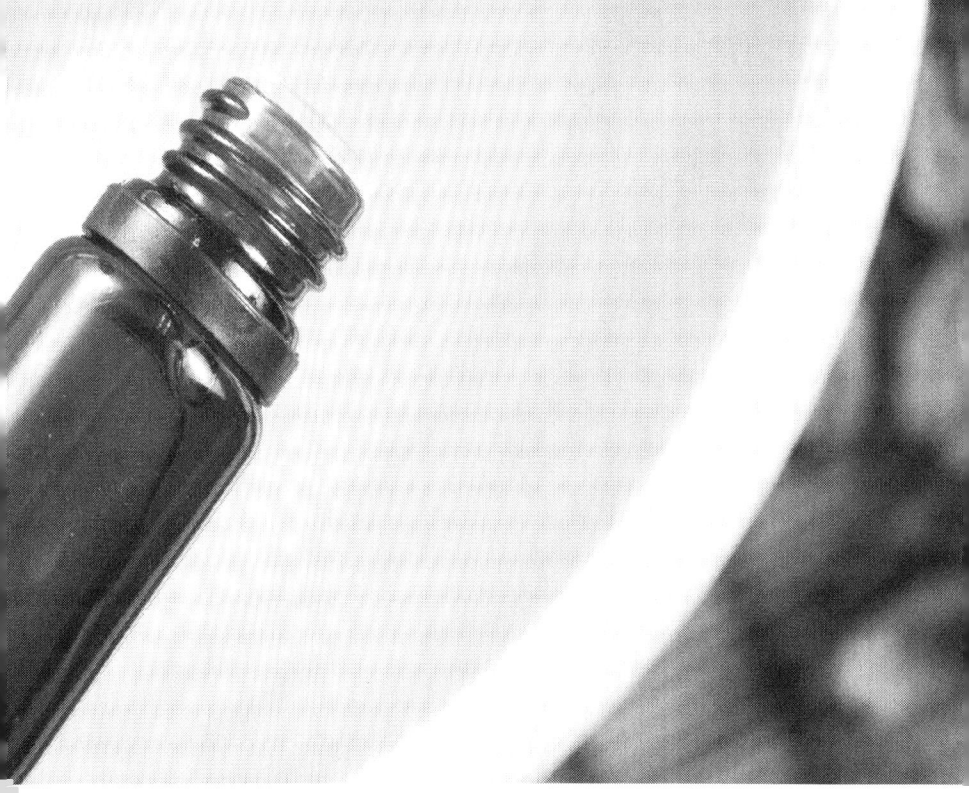

Spray Blends

Light Mist

This powerful mist is the one I use before and after each client session as well as when I travel, to clear hotel rooms of any unwanted energies. It raises the vibrational levels to create a more welcoming atmosphere anywhere and everywhere you are. This mist goes with me everywhere! I hope you love it as much as I do!

4 drops Sage EO (*Salvia officinalis*)
5 drops Lavender EO (*Lavendula angustifolia*)
1 Citrine chip
1 mini Selenite rod
1 Garnet chip
1 Amethyst chip
1 Black Tourmaline chip

Blend EOs and items together in a 1 oz spray bottle and fill to the shoulder with distilled or spring water.

Sage Mist

Use to cleanse an area, dwelling, object or otherwise, of unwanted energies; great for space clearings or before sacred practices. Spray around your body and environment liberally.

3 drops Sage EO (*Salvia officinalis*)
1 sprig White Mountain Sage
1 Citrine chip

Blend EOs and items together in a 1 oz spray bottle and fill to the shoulder with distilled or spring water.

Om It Out Spray

Use to enhance your meditation experience. Spray around your body and environment before your meditation sessions.

5 drops Ylang Ylang EO (*Cananga odorata*)
5 drops Rose Absolute (*Rosa damascena*)
4 drops Lavender EO (*Lavendula angustifolia*)
1 prong Star Anise
1 Garnet chip
1 Citrine chip
1 mini Selenite rod

Blend EOs and items together in a 1 oz spray bottle and fill to the shoulder with distilled or spring water.

Sweet Slumber Spray

Spray this on bed linen before sleeping each evening.

4 drops Lavender EO (*Lavendula angustifolia*)
1 drop Vanilla CO2 or Oleoresin (*Vanilla planifolia*)
1 Citrine chip

Blend EOs and items together in a 1 oz spray bottle and fill to the shoulder with distilled or spring water.

Violet Flame Spray

Channeled on September 24, 2010 – This spray invokes the power of St. Germaine to come in and plow the way clear for you and all your endeavors. [This batch makes four 1 oz bottles, or one 4 oz bottle.] Spray above head each morning to invoke St. Germaine and the Violet Flame into your day.

7 drops Ylang Ylang EO (*Cananga odorata*)
5 drops Jasmine Absolute (5%) (*Jasminum gradiflorum*)
9 drops Rosewood EO (*Aniba roseaodora*)
2 drops Rose Absolute (*Rosa damascena*)
3 drops Sandalwood EO (*Santalum album or S. paniculatum*)
1 drop Frankincense EO (*Boswellia carterii*)

Mix just the EOs into one bottle, swirl to blend together. Divide evenly into four 1 oz bottles; or you could create one 4 oz bottle, in which case you would not divide mixture. With EO blend in the bottle(s), add:

1 Garnet stone to each bottle
1 Citrine chip to each bottle

Fill to the shoulder with distilled or spring water.

REFRESHER MIST

This is my go to mist anytime I want a little pick me up during the day. Spray on skin, clothes, linens, and in any room or vehicle when you want a rich and uplifting scent.

6 drops Rosemary EO (*Rosmarinus officinalis*)
7 drops Peppermint EO (*Mentha piperita*)
1 Citrine chip
1 Clear Quartz chip

Blend EOs and items together in a 1 oz spray bottle and fill to the shoulder with distilled or spring water.

Orange Julius Mist

Love this funky, fresh scent that reminds me of one of my favorite childhood drinks, the Orange Julius. Spray liberally where ever you are guided to.

5 drops Sweet Orange EO (*Citrus sinensis*)
3 drops Vanilla CO2 or Oleoresin (*Vanilla planifolia*)
1 drop Peppermint EO (*Mentha piperita*)
1 Citrine chip

Blend EOs and items together in a 1 oz spray bottle and fill to the shoulder with distilled or spring water.

Recharging Spray

Anytime you would like a quick yet relaxing recharge during your day, spray this mist in the air and inhale deeply.

6 drops Rosemary EO (*Rosmarinus officinalis*)
4 drops Lavender EO (*Lavendula angustifolia*)
1 Citrine chip
1 Clear Quartz chip

Blend EOs and items together in a 1 oz spray bottle and fill to the shoulder with distilled or spring water.

Everyday Oil Blends

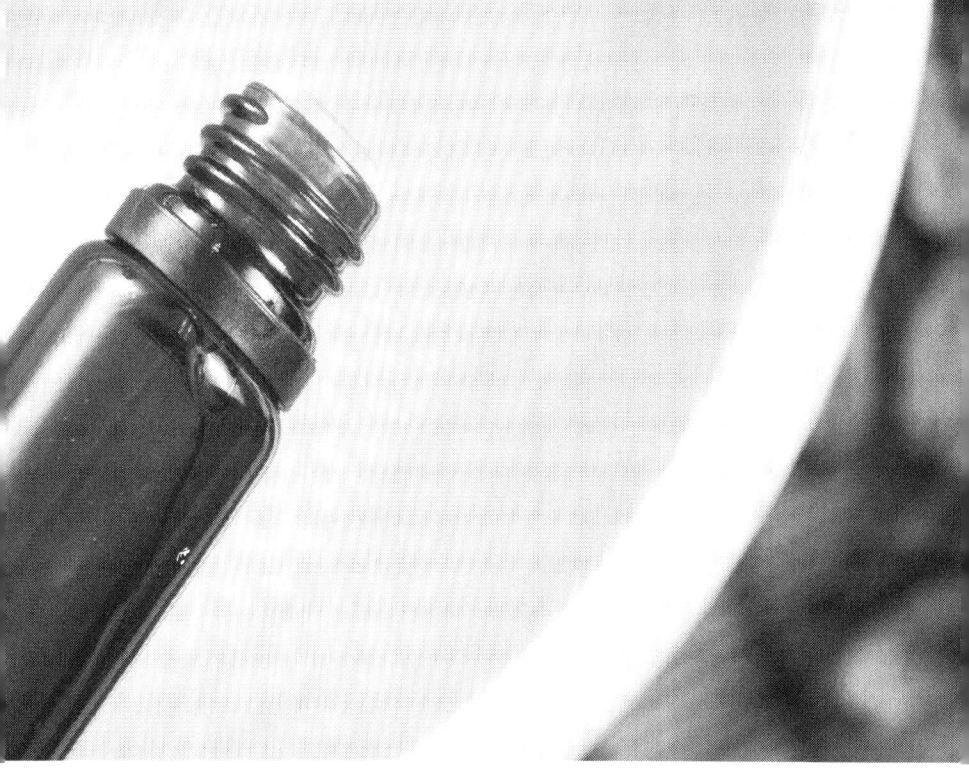

Flora's Signature Scent

I developed this blend in early 2004 and have worn it every day since! I hope you enjoy it as much as I do. Use liberally! Yay!

3 drops Bergamot EO (*Citrus bergamia*)
2 drops Lemongrass EO (*Cymbopogen citratus*)
1 drop Patchouli EO (*Pogostemon cablin*)
1 Citrine chip
1 mini Selenite rod
1 Amethyst chip

Blend EOs and items together in a 15ml dropper bottle and fill to the shoulder with your choice of carrier oil.

Angel Oil

Wear to connect with the Angelic Realm, your Guardian Angels or the Arch Angels. This blend was channeled in June of 2011.

3 drops Magnolia (*Michelia alba*) also known as White Champa Flower
3 drops Roman Chamomile EO (*Chamaemelum nobile*)
2 drops Jasmine Absolute (5%) (*Jasminum gradiflorum*)
3 drops Bergamot EO (*Citrus bergamia*)
1 drop Vanilla CO2 or Oleoresin (*Vanilla planifolia*)
1 Citrine chip
1 mini Selenite rod

Blend EOs and items together in a 15ml dropper bottle and fill to the shoulder with your choice of carrier oil.

Earth

Use this blend to connect with the energies of the element of Earth. This recipe was adapted from a recipe found in Scott Cunningham's "The Complete Book of Incense, Oils & Brews."

2 drops Patchouli EO (*Pogostemon cablin*)
1 drop Cypress EO (*Cupressus sempervirens*)
1 Citrine chip
1 tiny pebble from your land or a place that means a lot to you – thoroughly washed and dried

Blend EOs and items together in a 15ml dropper bottle and fill to the shoulder with your choice of carrier oil.

Water

Use this blend to connect with the energies of the element of Water. This recipe was adapted from a recipe found in Scott Cunningham's "The Complete Book of Incense, Oils & Brews."

1 drop Palmarosa EO (*Cymbopogen martini*)
1 drop Ylang Ylang EO (*Cananga odorata*)
1 drop Jasmine Absolute (5%) (*Jasminum gradiflorum*)
1 drop Magnolia EO (*Michelia alba*) also known as White Champa Flower
1 Citrine chip
1 Blue Topaz chip

Blend EOs and items together in a 15ml dropper bottle and fill to the shoulder with your choice of carrier oil.

AIR

Use this blend to connect with the energies of the element of Air. This recipe was adapted from a recipe found in Scott Cunningham's "The Complete Book of Incense, Oils & Brews."

2 drops Lavender EO (*Lavendula angustifolia*)
1 drop Sandalwood EO (*Santal album* or *Santal paniculatum*)
1 drop Neroli EO (*Citrus aurantium var amara*)
1 Citrine chip
1 mini Selenite rod

Blend EOs and items together in a 15ml dropper bottle and fill to the shoulder with your choice of carrier oil.

FIRE

Use this blend to connect with the energies of the element of Fire. This recipe was adapted from a recipe found in Scott Cunningham's "The Complete Book of Incense, Oils & Brews."

2 drops Ginger EO (*Zingiber officinale*)
2 drops Rosemary EO (*Rosmarinus officinalis*)
1 drop Clove EO (*Eugenia caryphyllata*)
1 drop Sweet Orange EO (*Citrus sinensis*)
1 Citrine chip
1 Red Jasper chip

Blend EOs and items together in a 15ml dropper bottle and fill to the shoulder with your choice of carrier oil.

Sun

Use this blend to connect with the Solar Energies.

3 drops Sweet Orange EO (*Citrus sinensis*)
1 drop Clove EO (*Eugenia caryophyllata*)
1 Citrine chip
1 Carnelian chip

Blend EOs and items together in a 15ml dropper bottle and fill to the shoulder with your choice of carrier oil.

Focus Formula Blend

Use this formula to bring about greater focus in your life. This works wonderfully before an exam, beginning a project or something you really want to focus on.

1 Green Aventurine chip
1 Black Tourmaline chip
1 Citrine chip

Fill vessel 2/3 full with the Air Elemental oil blend – for clear thinking and 1/3 full with the Earth Elemental oil blend – for grounding.

Blend oils and items together in a bottle size of your choosing. Tip several times to blend.

Third Eye

Use this blend to connect with the energies of the element of Spirit and to open your Third Eye area before ritual or any other psychic or divinatory endeavors.

3 drops Lemongrass EO (*Cymbopogon citratus*)
1 drop Cinnamon EO (*Cinnamomum zeylanicum*)
1 small piece Cinnamon Bark
1 mini Selenite rod
1 Citrine chip

Blend EOs and items together in a 15ml dropper bottle and fill to the shoulder with your choice of carrier oil.

Calming

Use this blend on your pulse points anytime you desire to bring calming energy into your space.

3 drops Lavender EO (*Lavendula angustifolia*)
2 drops Rosewood EO (*Aniba roseaodora*)
1 Citrine chip
1 Rose Quartz chip
1 Amethyst chip

Blend EOs and items together in a 15ml dropper bottle and fill to the shoulder with your choice of carrier oil.

"YipYip" Ritual Preparation Oil

This oil was inspired by the 2010 Z. Budapest Goddess Festival. Adorn yourself before ritual with this Goddess inspired oil! Yay!!!

3 drops Lemongrass EO (*Cymbopogon citratus*)
2 drops Peppermint EO (*Mentha piperita*)
2 drops Sage EO (*Salvia officinalis*)
1 small piece of White Mountain Sage Stick [only the stick]
1 small piece Blond Sandalwood
1 whole Clove with top
1 Citrine chip
1 mini Selenite rod

Blend EOs and items together in a 15ml dropper bottle and fill to the shoulder with your choice of carrier oil.

Money Draw Oil

Use this to anoint your purse, wallet, debit cards, paper money and coins to bring in more prosperity each time you spend.

3 drop Patchouli EO (*Pogostemon cablin*)
1 Peridot chip
1 Citrine chip

Blend EOs and items together in a 15ml dropper bottle and fill to the shoulder with your choice of carrier oil.

Massage Blends

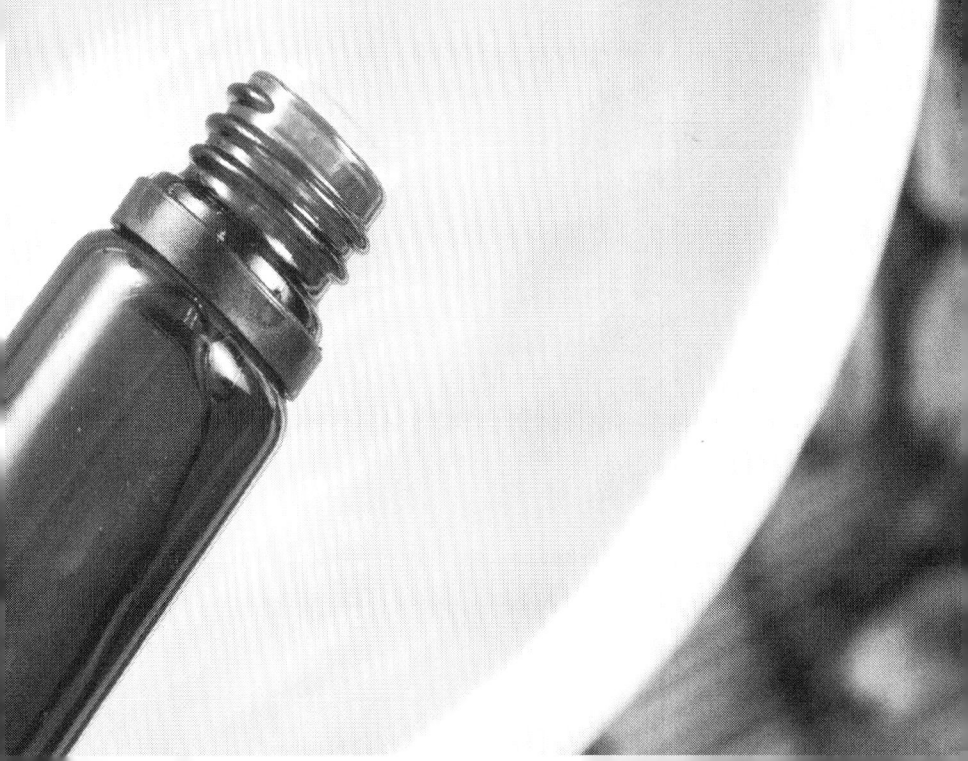

Spa Getaway Blend

Need a getaway? This blend will be sure to take your mind off of your current issues and transport you to your personal Spa Getaway!

9 drops Sweet Orange EO (*Citrus sinensis*)
5 drops Ginger EO (*Zingiber officinale*)
2 drops Lavender EO (*Lavendula angustifolia*)

Add the EO's to a 2 oz bottle of carrier oil, close and gently shake to blend the oils. Use all over your body for that getaway feeling.

Energy Blend

Need more energy? This blend will surely do the trick!

3 drops Bergamot EO (*Citrus bergamia*)
3 drops Rosemary EO (*Rosemarinus officinalis ct. camphor*)
3 drops Grapefruit EO (*Citrus paradisi*)
3 drops Lemon EO (*Citrus limon*)
3 drops Orange EO (*Citrus sinensis*)
3 drops Basil EO (*Ocimum basilicum ct. linalool*)

Add the EO's to a 2 oz bottle of carrier oil, close and gently shake to blend the oils. Use on pulse points when you need a boost.

Do not apply just before going out into the sun, or keep the area covered, as some of the citrus oils in this recipe can be phototoxic.

Headache Blend

Massage liberally on base of neck and temples when you have a headache.

9 drops Sweet Marjoram EO (*Marjorana origanum*)
9 drops Peppermint EO (*Mentha piperita*)

Add the EO's to a 2 oz bottle of carrier oil, close and gently shake to blend the oils.

Lymphatic Massage Blend

This blend is one I have been using for many many years. This blend is great for detoxifying the lymph nodes, liver, reduce water retention and improve your immunity.

8 drops Lemon EO (*Citrus limon*)
8 drops Grapefruit EO (*Citrus paradisi*)
6 drops Rosemary EO (*Rosemarinus officinalis*)
4 drops Juniper Berry EO (optional) (*Juniperus communis*)

Add the EO's to a 2 oz bottle of carrier oil, close and gently shake to blend the oils. Use liberally.

Foot Restore Blend

Massage liberally on feet when you need to restore them from too much standing, for achiness or overall generally tired feet.

10 drops Peppermint EO (*Mentha piperita*)
6 drops Eucalyptus EO (*Eucalyptus globulus*)

Add the EO's to a 2 oz bottle of carrier oil, close and gently shake to blend the oils.

FIVE STAR HOTEL BLEND

Massage liberally over hands, feet and joints to relax every nerve ending. This will surely bring you to a place of rest and relaxation.

8 drops Lavender EO (*Lavendula angustifolia*)
6 drops Vanilla CO2 or Oleoresin (*Vanilla planifolia*)

Add the EO's to a 2 oz bottle of carrier oil, close and gently shake to blend the oils.

DEEP SLEEP BLEND

Massage liberally over feet before bedtime. This will surely bring you to a place of deep sleep and relaxation.

6 drops Valerian EO (*Valeriana officinalis*)
2 drops Lavender EO (*Lavendula angustifolia*)

Add the EO's to a 2 oz bottle of carrier oil, close and gently shake to blend the oils.

Chakra Oils

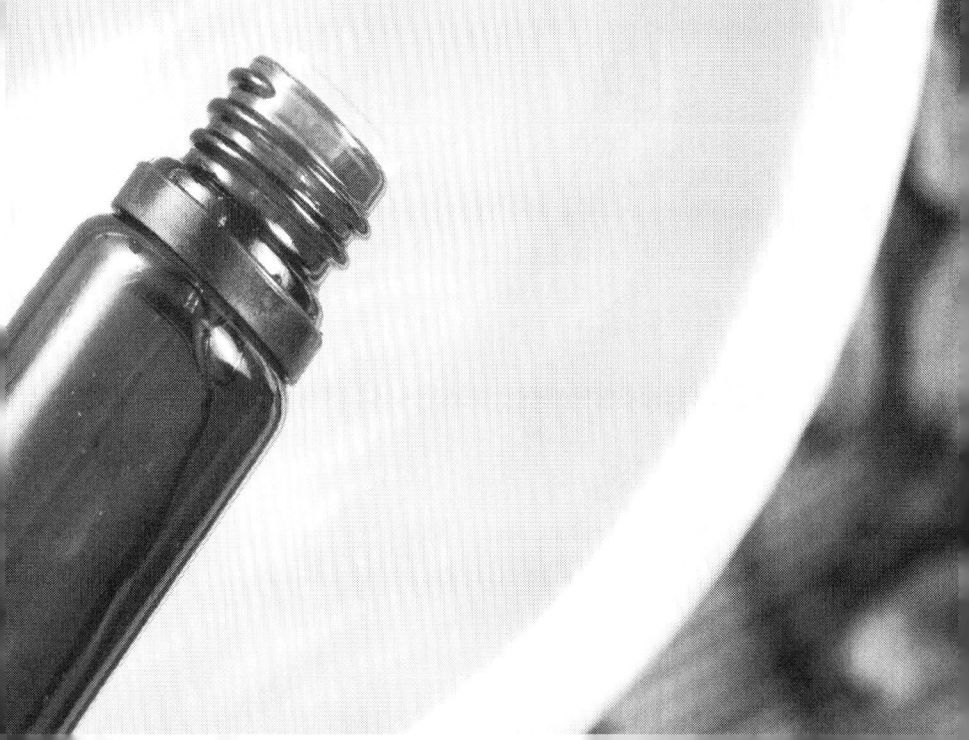

Chakras or Energy Centers in the body should be balanced and harmonized every day. While the body has thousands of Chakras this section focuses on the 11 main energy centers.

Anoint each Chakra point starting from the root Chakra going up. As you anoint each point envision that area illuminating with bright, radiant light, and universal source energy.

Meditate on opening up the Chakra areas and releasing any blockages. Once all are clear, fill with universal light and energy, and then close. This will keep the Chakras clear and in working order. Repeat daily.

Earth Star Chakra

Location ~ About six inches below your feet
Color ~ Shades of Black – Or your personal color of strength for this Chakra
1 Black & Brown Tourmaline chip
3 drops Ginger EO (*Zingiber officinale*)

Blend EO and crystal together in a 15ml dropper bottle and fill to the shoulder with your choice of carrier oil. To store, wrap in a cloth of the corresponding color.

Root Chakra

Location ~ Base of spine in the area of the lumbar
Color ~ Red – Or your personal color of strength for this Chakra
1 Garnet chip
3 drops Patchouli EO (*Pogostemon cablin*)

Blend EO and crystal together in a 15ml dropper bottle and fill to the shoulder with your choice of carrier oil. To store, wrap in a cloth of the corresponding color.

SACRAL CHAKRA

Location ~ The area 1" to 2" below the navel
Color ~ Orange – Or your personal color of strength for this Chakra
1 Carnelian chip
3 drops Sweet Orange EO (*Citrus sinensis*)

Blend EO and crystal together in a 15ml dropper bottle and fill to the shoulder with your choice of carrier oil. To store, wrap in a cloth of the corresponding color.

SOLAR PLEXUS CHAKRA

Location ~ One hand width up from the navel
Color ~ Yellow – Or your personal color of strength for this Chakra
1 Citrine chip
3 drops Lemongrass EO (*Cymbopogon citratus*)

Blend EO and crystal together in a 15ml dropper bottle and fill to the shoulder with your choice of carrier oil. To store, wrap in a cloth of the corresponding color.

HEART CHAKRA

Location ~ Behind breast bone
Color ~ Green – Or your personal color of strength for this Chakra
1 Peridot chip
3 drops Eucalyptus EO (*Eucalyptus globulus*)

Blend EO and crystal together in a 15ml dropper bottle and fill to the shoulder with your choice of carrier oil. To store, wrap in a cloth of the corresponding color.

HIGHER HEART CHAKRA – SELF LOVE/UNCONDITIONAL LOVE

Location ~ Half of a hand width above breast bone
Color ~ Pink – Or your personal color of strength for this Chakra
1 Rose Quartz chip
3 drops Rose Absolute (*Rosa damascena*)

Blend EO and crystal together in a 15ml dropper bottle and fill to the shoulder with your choice of carrier oil. To store, wrap in a cloth of the corresponding color.

THROAT CHAKRA

Location ~ Center of neck
Color ~ Blue – Or your personal color of strength for this Chakra
1 Blue Topaz chip
3 drops Geranium EO (*Pelargonium graveolens*)

Blend EO and crystal together in a 15ml dropper bottle and fill to the shoulder with your choice of carrier oil. To store, wrap in a cloth of the corresponding color.

INNER THROAT CHAKRA

Location ~ Inside voice box
Color ~ Turquoise – Or your personal color of strength for this

Chakra
1 Turquoise chip
3 drops Clary Sage EO (*Salvia sclarea*)

Blend EO and crystal together in a 15ml dropper bottle and fill to the shoulder with your choice of carrier oil. To store, wrap in a cloth of the corresponding color.

BROW CHAKRA

Location ~ Between eyebrows and slightly up on the forehead
Color ~ Indigo – Or your personal color of strength for this Chakra
1 Amethyst chip
3 drops Bergamot EO (*Citrus bergamia*)

Blend EO and crystal together in a 15ml dropper bottle and fill to the shoulder with your choice of carrier oil. To store, wrap in a cloth of the corresponding color.

CROWN CHAKRA

Location ~ Top back of head
Color ~ Violet – Or your personal color of strength for this Chakra
1 Clear Quartz chip
3 drops Lavender EO (*Lavendula angustifolia*)

Blend EO and crystal together in a 15ml dropper bottle and fill to the shoulder with your choice of carrier oil. To store, wrap in a cloth of the corresponding color.

Soul Star Chakra

Location ~ About 6" to 12" above head
Color ~ White Iridescent Light – Or your personal color of strength for this Chakra
1 mini Selenite rod
3 drops Jasmine Absolute (5%) (*Jasminum gradiflorum*)

Blend EO and crystal together in a 15ml dropper bottle and fill to the shoulder with your choice of carrier oil. To store, wrap in a cloth of the corresponding color.

For more information regarding Chakras:

CLASSES:
The Body's Energy Centers – Chakras 101
&
Color Therapy
http://www.mflorapeterson-innercircle.com/shop/classes/

MEDITATIONS:
Chakra Balancing and Cleansing Meditation
http://www.mflorapeterson-innercircle.com/shop/meditations/

Solar Cycle Blends

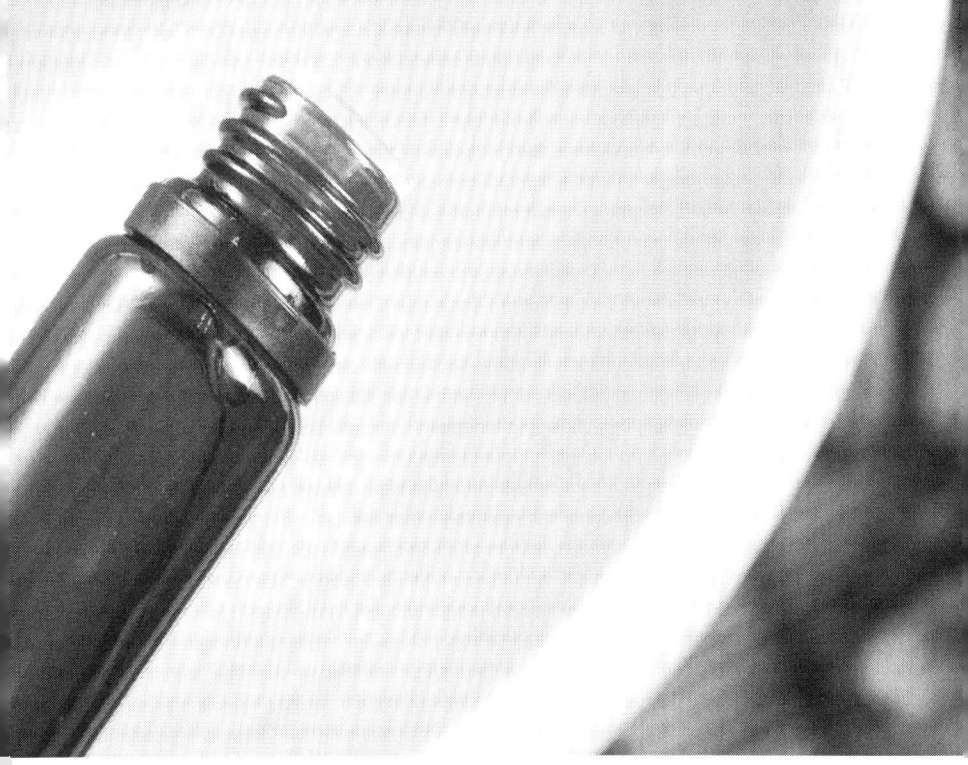

Every six weeks the sun enters into a new cycle or phase. These solar cycles are sometimes called Sabbats. People who honor Sabbats often celebrate these cycles with celebrations, food, drink and merriment. These celebrations can last all week, all day, an hour or for a few minutes, and are conducted in a ritual circle or special sacred space. These solar cycle blends can be used anytime during the year to connect with the energies of the sun and the cycle that it is in.

The Solar Wheel of the Year
Northern Hemisphere

- Yule/Winter Solstice — December 21-23
- Candlemas/Imbolc — February 2
- Ostara/Spring Equinox — March 21-23
- Beltane/May Day — May 1
- Summer Solstice/Litha — June 21-23
- Lammas — August 1
- Mabon/Fall Equinox — September 21-23
- Samhain/Halloween — October 31

Southern Hemisphere

- Yule/Winter Solstice — June 21-23
- Candlemas/Imbolc — August 1
- Ostara/Spring Equinox — September 21-23
- Beltane/May Day — October 31
- Summer Solstice/Litha — December 21-23
- Lammas — February 2
- Mabon/Fall Equinox — March 21-23
- Samhain/Halloween — May 1

Winter Solstice / Yule

3 drops Rosemary EO (*Rosemarinus officinalis ct. camphor*)
2 drops Frankincense EO (*Boswellia carterii*)
1 drop Sandalwood EO (*Santalum album or S. paniculatum*)
1 Pine Needle
1 Citrine chip

Blend EOs and items together in a 15ml dropper bottle and fill to the shoulder with your choice of carrier oil.

Candlemas / Imbolc

3 drops Basil EO (*Ocimum basilicum*)
3 drops Peppermint EO (*Mentha piperita*)
3 drops Rosemary EO (*Rosemarinus officinalis ct. camphor*)
1 small piece White Mountain Sage
1 Citrine chip

Blend EOs and items together in a 15ml dropper bottle and fill to the shoulder with your choice of carrier oil.

Ostara / Spring Equinox

3 drops of Rose Absolute (*Rosa damascena*)
3 drops Jasmine Absolute (5%) (*Jasminum gradiflorum*)
1 drop of Sandalwood EO (*Santalum album or S. paniculatum*)
1 Citrine chip

Blend EOs and items together in a 15ml dropper bottle and fill to the shoulder with your choice of carrier oil.

Beltane / May Day

2 drops Rosewood EO (*Aniba rosaeodora*)
2 drops Rosemary EO (*Rosemarinus officinalis ct. camphor*)
2 drops Geranium EO (*Pelargonium graveolens*)
2 drops Rose Absolute (*Rosa damascena*)
1 Citrine chip

Blend EOs and items together in a 15ml dropper bottle and fill to the shoulder with your choice of carrier oil.

Summer Solstice / Litha

3 drops Sweet Orange EO (*Citrus sinensis*)
3 drops Ginger EO (*Zingiber officinale*)
2 drops Peppermint EO (*Mentha piperita*)
1 Citrine chip

Blend EOs and items together in a 15ml dropper bottle and fill to the shoulder with your choice of carrier oil.

Lammas

2 drops of Patchouli EO (*Pogostemon cablin*)
1 drop Rosemary EO (*Rosemarinus officinalis ct. camphor*)
1 piece Blond Sandalwood
1 Citrine chip

Blend EOs and items together in a 15ml dropper bottle and fill to the shoulder with your choice of carrier oil.

Mabon / Fall Equinox

6 drops Sage EO (*Salvia officinalis*)
5 drops Patchouli EO (*Pogostemon cablin*)
3 drops Myrrh EO (*Commiphora myrrha*)
2 drops Rose Absolute (*Rosa damascena*)
1 small piece White Mountain Sage
1 Citrine chip

Blend EOs and items together in a 15ml dropper bottle and fill to the shoulder with your choice of carrier oil.

Samhain / Halloween

2 drops Sage EO (*Salvia officinalis*)
2 drops Patchouli EO (*Pogostemon cablin*)
2 drops Sweet Orange EO (*Citrus sinensis*)
1 Citrine chip

Blend EOs and items together in a 15ml dropper bottle and fill to the shoulder with your choice of carrier oil.

Lunar Cycle Blends

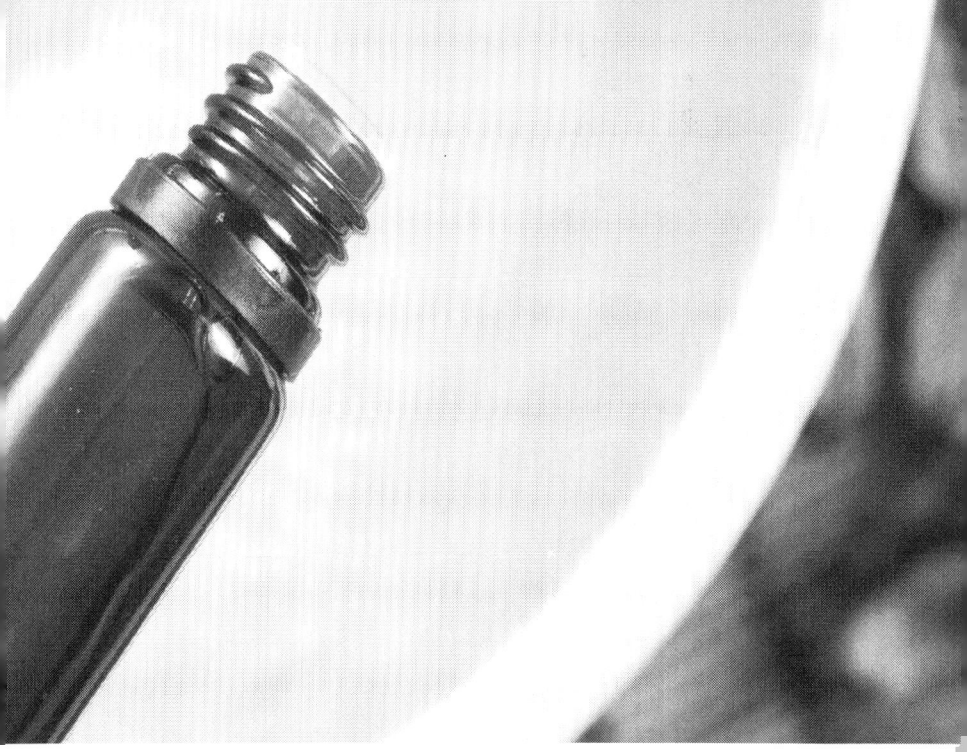

Honoring the Moon and Her Influences

Mother Nature as well as the body's our Spirits are housed in, are all influenced by the Moons pull on water. When we connect with the Moons energy daily, we tune into the ebb and flow of energy within us as well as without, just like the ebb and flow of the Oceans tides.

Use the oils liberally when you want to connect with the aspects and energies of the Moon.

Full Moon – [2 days before, the day of the Full Moon & 2 days after]

2 drops Rosewood EO (*Aniba roseaodora*)
2 drops Jasmine Absolute (5%) (*Jasminum gradiflorum*)
1 Moonstone chip
1 Citrine chip

Blend EOs and items together in a 15ml dropper bottle and fill to the shoulder with your choice of carrier oil.

New Moon – [New Moon – the first quarter]

3 drops Bergamot EO (*Citrus bergamia*)
2 drops Magnolia EO (*Michelia alba*) aka. White Champa Flower
1 Dark Moonstone chip
1 Black Tourmaline chip
1 mini Selenite rod
1 Citrine chip

Blend EOs and items together in a 15ml dropper bottle and fill to the shoulder with your choice of carrier oil.

DARK MOON — [25 – 28 DAYS AFTER THE NEW MOON]

3 drops Bergamot EO (*Citrus bergamia*)
1 drop Frankincense EO (*Boswellia carterii*)
1 Dark Moonstone chip
1 Black Tourmaline chip
1 Citrine chip

Blend EOs and items together in a 15ml dropper bottle and fill to the shoulder with your choice of carrier oil.

BLUE MOON — [THE SECOND FULL MOON IN ONE MONTH OR THE FOURTH FULL MOON IN A QUARTER — BASED ON THE SOLAR CYCLES]

3 drops Roman Chamomile EO (*Chamaemelum nobile*)
3 drops Jasmine Absolute (5%) (*Jasminum gradiflorum*)
1 Rainbow Moonstone chip
1 Labradorite chip
1 Citrine chip

Blend EOs and items together in a 15ml dropper bottle and fill to the shoulder with your choice of carrier oil.

PURPLE MOON — [THE SECOND NEW MOON IN ONE MONTH OR THE FOURTH NEW MOON IN A QUARTER — BASED ON THE SOLAR CYCLES]

3 drops Bergamot EO (*Citrus bergamia*)
2 drops Heather Absolute (*Calluna vulgaris*)
1 Brown Tourmaline chip
1 Black Tourmaline chip
1 Purple Fluorite chip

1 Amethyst chip
1 Citrine chip

Blend EOs and items together in a 15ml dropper bottle and fill to the shoulder with your choice of carrier oil.

Lotion Blends

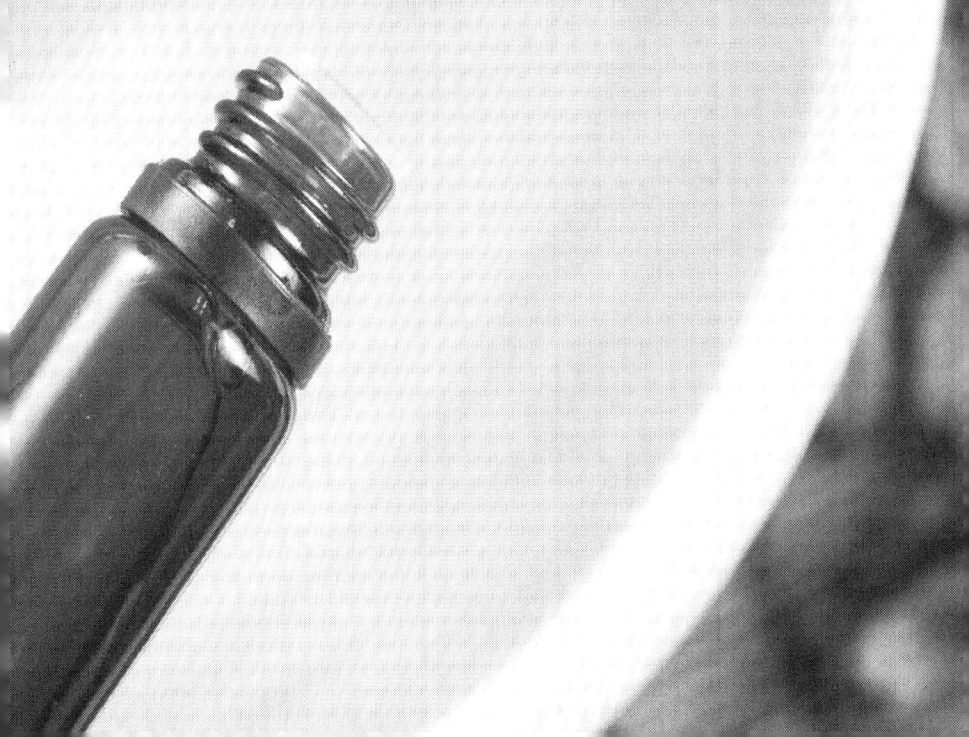

Lymphatic Message Lotion Blend

This blend is one I have been using for many years. This blend is great for detoxifying the lymph nodes, liver, reduce water retention and improve your immunity.

8 drops Lemon EO (*Citrus limon*)
8 drops Grapefruit EO (*Citrus paradisi*)
6 drops Rosemary EO (*Rosemarinus officinalis ct. camphor*)

Add the EO's to a 4 oz jar filled with unscented lotion of your choice, stir thoroughly to blend the oils and lotion. Use liberally.

Energy Lotion Blend

Need more energy? This blend will surely do the trick!

3 drops Bergamot EO (*Citrus bergamia*)
3 drops Rosemary EO (*Rosemarinus officinalis ct. camphor*)
3 drops Grapefruit EO (*Citrus paradisi*)
3 drops Lemon EO (*Citrus limon*)
3 drops Sweet Orange EO (*Citrus sinensis*)
3 drops Basil EO (*Basilcum ocimum*)

Add the EO's to a 4 oz jar filled with unscented lotion of your choice, stir thoroughly to blend the oils and lotion. Use liberally anytime you would like to experience more energy.

Headache Lotion Blend

Massage liberally on base of neck and temples when you have a headache.

9 drops Lavender EO (*Lavendula angustifolia*)
9 drops Peppermint EO (*Mentha piperita*)
3 drops Sweet Marjoram EO (*Origanum marjorana*)

Add the EO's to a 4 oz jar filled with unscented lotion of your choice, stir thoroughly to blend the oils and lotion. Use liberally.

Spa Getaway Lotion Blend

Need a getaway? This blend will be sure to take your mind off of your current issues and transport you to your personal Spa Getaway!

9 drops Sweet Orange EO (*Citrus sinensis*)
5 drops Ginger EO (*Zingiber officinale*)
3 drops Lavender EO (*Lavendula angustifolia*)

Add the EO's to a 4 oz jar filled with unscented lotion of your choice, stir thoroughly to blend the oils and lotion. Use liberally. Use all over your body for that getaway feeling.

Foot Restore Lotion Blend

Massage liberally on feet when you need to restore them from too much standing, for achiness or overall generally tired feet.

10 drops Peppermint EO (*Mentha piperita*)
6 drops Eucalyptus EO (*Eucalyptus globulus*)
1 drop Lavender EO (*Lavendula angustifolia*)

Add the EO's to a 4 oz jar filled with unscented lotion of your choice, stir thoroughly to blend the oils and lotion. Use liberally.

FIVE STAR HOTEL LOTION BLEND

Massage liberally over hands, feet and joints to relax every nerve ending. This will surely bring you to a place of rest and relaxation.

8 drops Lavender EO (*Lavendula angustifolia*)
6 drops Vanilla CO2 or Oleoresin (*Vanilla planifolia*)

Add the EO's to a 4 oz jar filled with unscented lotion of your choice, stir thoroughly to blend the oils and lotion. Use liberally.

COOL BREEZES LOTION

5 drops Lavender EO (*Lavendula angustifolia*)
5 drops Peppermint EO (*Mentha piperita*)
5 drops Ylang-Ylang EO (*Cananga odorata*)

Add the EO's to a 4 oz jar filled with unscented lotion of your choice, stir thoroughly to blend the oils and lotion. Use liberally anytime you want to feel to cool breeze of summer.

EARTH SECRETS LOTION

10 drops Sandalwood EO (*Santalum album or S. paniculatum*)
3 drops Patchouli EO (*Pogostemon cablin*)
3 drops Frankincense EO (*Boswellia carterii*)
1 drop Jasmine Absolute (5%) (*Jasminum gradiflorum*)

Add the EO's to a 4 oz jar filled with unscented lotion of your choice, stir thoroughly to blend the oils and lotion. Use liberally anytime you want to relax.

Sweet Slumber Lotion Blend

5 drops Lavender EO (*Lavendula angustifolia*)
2 drop Vanilla CO2 or Oleoresin (*Vanilla planifolia*)

Add the EO's to a 4 oz jar filled with unscented lotion of your choice, stir thoroughly to blend the oils and lotion. Use liberally before bedtime.

Lavender Lotion

5 drops Lavender EO (*Lavendula angustifolia*)

Add the EO's to a 4 oz jar filled with unscented lotion of your choice, stir thoroughly to blend the oils and lotion. Use liberally anytime you want to relax.

Vanilla Dream Lotion

8 drops Vanilla CO2 or Oleoresin (*Vanilla planifolia*)

Add the EO's to a 4 oz jar filled with unscented lotion of your choice, stir thoroughly to blend the oils and lotion. Use liberally anytime you want to relax.

Deep Sleep Blend

8 drops Valerian EO (*Valeriana officinalis*)
3 drops Lavender EO (*Lavendula angustifolia*)

Add the EO's to a 4 oz jar filled with unscented lotion of your choice, stir thoroughly to blend the oils and lotion. Massage liberally over feet before bedtime. This will surely bring you to a place of deep sleep and relaxation.

How to Create Your Own Blends

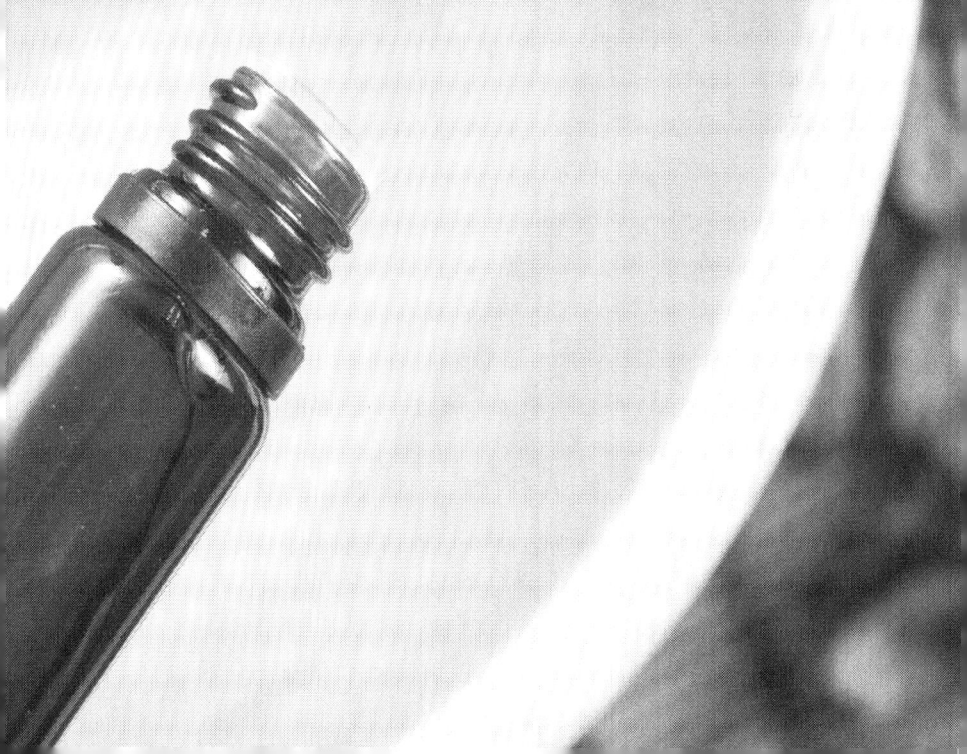

What Blends Well Together?

Creating your own blends may sound a bit daunting, but once you get started you will soon realize there are endless possibilities. There are a few schools of thought when it comes to blending oils: the first being to blend them by Group, Effect and Note. The second is to blend them intuitively. I tend to blend by intuition but the choice is up to you.

Let me explain a bit about Group, Effect and Note for you, each of these plays a different role in your blend and on the senses.

The Group

When blending, sometimes it is helpful to know what Group you would like to pick your Essential Oil from.

- Flowers
- Resins
- Trees
- Citrus
- Exotics
- Herbs
- Spices

If you generally like spicy scents, then I recommend choosing your oil from the Spice Group. If you like floral, then choose from the Flowers Group. It's really quite intuitive.

Most Essential Oils found in the same Group typically blends quite nicely together. However, floral scents also blend well with Citrus as well as Herbal.

One way to see what your nose thinks of the scents together is to open the bottles, hold them with one hand and waft them under your nose as you inhale with your eyes closed. This will give you a general idea of what they will smell like if blended together.

The Effect

Every plant, spice, fruit, flower, root, resin and so on has its own essence, energy, vibration and its own medicinal properties to take into account. Effects are also broken down into two main classes: Calming or Stimulating. It is best to look at the intention of your blend and then choose from one of the two Effects.

Calming includes the following Effects:

- Grounding
- Balancing
- Soothing
- Relaxing
- Supportive
- Sedating, etc…

Stimulating includes the following Effects:

- Lively
- Uplifting
- Refreshing
- Upbeat
- Energizing
- Warm
- Invigorating, etc…

It's recommend that you stay within the Effect that you intend for the blend; however, I have many blends that have Essential Oils from both Effects that work quite nicely.

The Note

The last thing to keep in mind when blending is to look at the Note of the Essential Oil. As in music, certain notes blend well with other notes and some notes may not blend so nicely together. The same holds true with Essential Oil blends.

There are three distinct Notes: Top, Middle and Base.

Top Notes

The first smell to arise from a blend and evaporate quickly. The top note fragrance is usually light, fresh, sharp, penetrating and airy. They add brightness and create the first impressions of your blend. The aroma of top note oils reminds me of wind chimes or a flute. Top notes stimulate and clear your mind and are uplifting to your energy.

Examples: Lemon, Grapefruit, Bergamot and Sweet Orange.

Middle Note

Called the "heart" note, these oils give the blend softness, fullness, and can round off any sharp edges. Middle notes can have both top and base note aromas within them. They are harmonizing for your blends – middle notes provide balance both physically and energetically. They are soothing and harmonizing for the mind and body.

Examples: German Chamomile, Roman Chamomile, Eucalyptus, Geranium, Helichrysum, Lavender, Lemongrass, Marjoram, Ravintsara, Rosemary, and Tea Tree.

Base Note

These oils provide a deep, warm, grounded quality to your blend. They function as "fixatives" and help reduce the evaporation of top notes. Base notes add intensity to a blend and often have an earthy aroma. The aroma rises slowly to your nose, unlike top notes, which penetrate quickly. Base notes are used to relieve stress, anxiety, and insomnia. They are calming and grounding. Most oils derived from woods, resins, and roots are base notes. Some of these oils can actually improve with age.

Examples: Frankincense, Patchouli, Sandalwood, Spikenard, Vetiver, and Ylang Ylang.

When blending, try to add one drop at a time to your blend, then mix and smell. Allow the blend to unfold slowly and inform you about what oils to add and how much. We often need much less essential oil than we might imagine.

Remember to keep track of the blends you make as you make them, so if you like them you can recreate them in the future. For example make note of the number of drops of Essential Oils you use as well as the type of oil in the blend, the date and time you created it and any other information you would like to note to yourself. There are worksheets in the back of this book to help you keep track of your unique blends.

Source for Notes: http://www.AromaticWisdomInstitute.com

Essential Oil Attributes

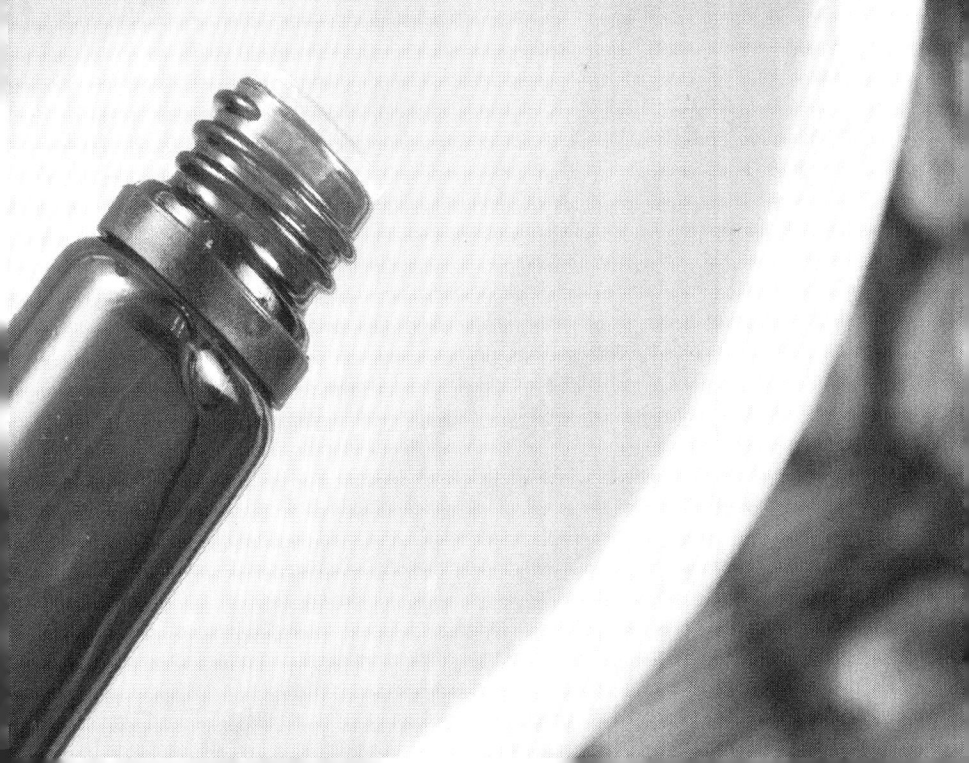

Citrus

- Bergamot – Top – Stimulating, Calming, Balancing depending on amount used
- Citronella – Top & Middle – Soothing
- Grapefruit – Top – Stimulating, Refreshing, Uplifting
- Lemon – Top - Stimulating, Refreshing
- Lemongrass – Top & Middle - Sedating, Soothing
- Lime – Top – Uplifting
- Mandarin – Top – Calming
- Sweet Orange – Top – Calming, Relaxing, Refreshing, Lively, Upbeat, Balancing, depending on amount used
- Tangerine – Top – Calming, Sedative, Soothing, Cheerful
- Verbena – Top & Middle - Stimulating

Herbs

- Angelica – Top - Stimulating
- Basil – Top & Middle - Stimulating
- Carrot Seed – Middle - Stimulating
- Celery – Top & Middle - Stimulating
- Clary Sage – Top & Middle – Calming, Balancing
- Dill – Middle - Stimulating
- Fennel – Top & Middle – Stimulating, Energizing
- Hyssop – Middle – Sedative, Stimulating, Balancing
- Sweet Marjoram – Middle – Calming, Sedating
- Peppermint – Top & Middle – Stimulating, Energy
- Rosemary – Middle - Stimulating
- Spearmint – Top – Calming, Stimulating
- Thyme – Middle – Stimulating, Energizing

Flowers

- Chamomile – Top & Middle – Calming, Sedative
- Geranium – Middle – Stimulating, Balancing, Sedative, depending on amount used
- Jasmine Absolute – Middle & Base – Sedative, Relaxant
- Lavender – Top & Middle – Relaxing, Stimulant depending on amount used
- Neroli – Middle – Calming, soothing, Relaxing, Uplifting, Balancing
- Rose Absolute – Middle & Base – Calming, Supportive
- Violet – Middle – Calming, Balancing

Trees

- Cedar Wood – Middle & Base – Calming, Grounding, Balancing
- Cypress – Middle & Base – comforting, soothing
- Eucalyptus – Top - Stimulating
- Juniper – Top & Middle - Stimulating
- Myrtle – Middle - Stimulating
- Petigrain – Top & Middle – Calming, Sedating
- Pine – Middle - Invigorating
- Rosewood – Middle & Base – Calming, Relaxing
- Tea Tree – Top & Middle - Stimulating

Exotics

- Palmarose – Middle – Uplifting, Rejuvenating
- Patchouli – Base – Sedating, Stimulating, depending on amount used
- Sandalwood – Base – Relaxing, Balancing, Grounding

- Vetiver – Base – Grounding, Balancing, Relaxing, Sedating
- YlangYlang – Middle & Base – Relaxing

Resins

- Benzoin – Base - Grounding
- Camphor – Base – Stimulating, Balancing
- Fir Needle – Middle - Grounding
- Frankincense – Base – Calming, Centering
- Myrrh – Base – Grounding, Stimulating
- Vanilla Absolute – Base - Calming

Spices

- Aniseed – Top & Middle - Stimulating
- Bay – Top & Middle - Stimulating
- Black Pepper – Middle – Stimulating, Grounding
- Cardamom – Top & Middle - Stimulating
- Cinnamon – Middle & Base – Invigorating, Warm
- Clove – Middle & Base – Stimulating, Energizing
- Coriander – Top – Stimulating, Uplifting
- Ginger – Middle & Base - Stimulating
- Nutmeg – Middle – Calming, Sedating

Source: http://www.serenearomatherapy.com/essential-oil-blend.html

Your Essential Oil Worksheet Pages

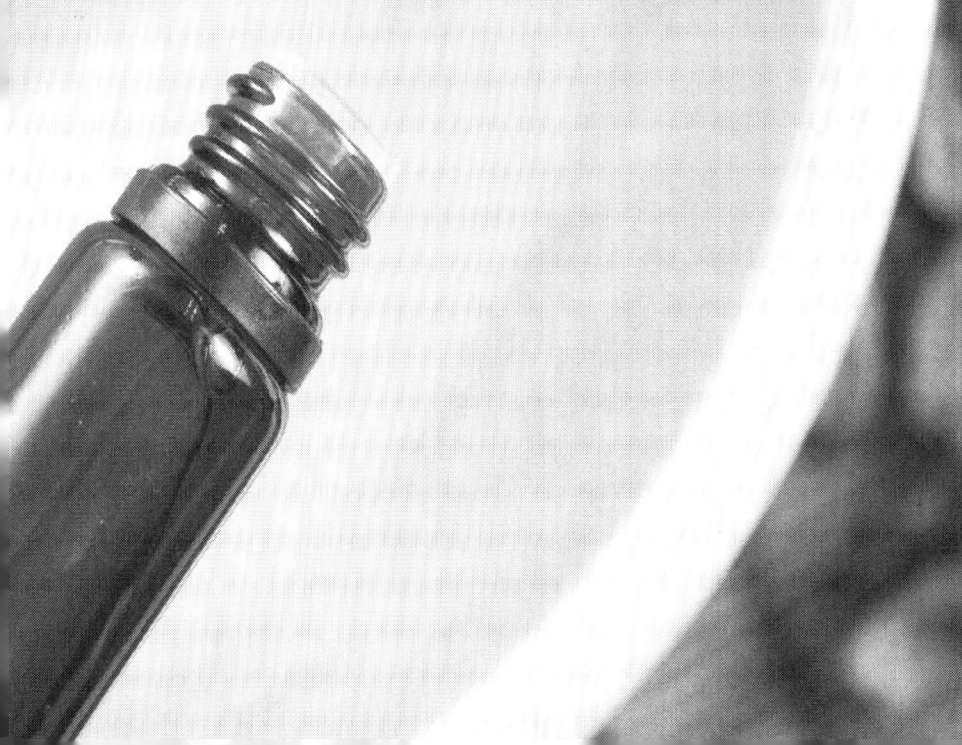

Your Essential Oil Recipe Blends, Worksheets, and notes pages

Scribbling down notes on small pieces of paper throughout my day about scents that I loved and ideas of what other scents they might blend well with is how I started blending and making my recipes. Many times I would want to recreate those blends and found myself digging in all the nooks and crannies of my sacred space room to find those slips of paper.

Here you have ample room to scribble to your heart's content and create your own Essential Oil blends based on your personal and Spiritual needs.

Happy blending!

My Own Essential Oil Recipe Blend

Date:_____

Name of blend:_____

Size vessel:_____

Carrier oil: _____

Essential oil: _____

Essential oil: _____

Essential oil: _____

Essential oil: _____

Essential oil: _____

Crystal: _____

Other items:_____

Notes about blend:_____

_____

_____

_____

_____

_____

My Own Essential Oil Recipe Blend

Date:_____

Name of blend:_____

Size vessel:_____

Carrier oil:_____

Essential oil:_____

Essential oil:_____

Essential oil:_____

Essential oil:_____

Essential oil:_____

Crystal:_____

Other items:_____

Notes about blend:_____

_____

_____

_____

_____

_____

My Own Essential Oil Recipe Blend

Date:_____

Name of blend:_____

Size vessel:_____

Carrier oil: _____

Essential oil: _____

Essential oil: _____

Essential oil: _____

Essential oil: _____

Essential oil: _____

Crystal: _____

Other items:_____

Notes about blend:_____

_____

_____

_____

_____

_____

My Own Essential Oil Recipe Blend

Date:_____

Name of blend:_____

Size vessel:_____

Carrier oil:_____

Essential oil:_____

Essential oil:_____

Essential oil:_____

Essential oil:_____

Essential oil:_____

Crystal:_____

Other items:_____

Notes about blend:_____

_____

_____

_____

_____

_____

My Own Essential Oil Recipe Blend

Date:_____

Name of blend:_____

Size vessel:_____

Carrier oil: _____

Essential oil: _____

Essential oil: _____

Essential oil: _____

Essential oil: _____

Essential oil: _____

Crystal: _____

Other items:_____

Notes about blend:_____

_____

_____

_____

_____

_____

My Own Essential Oil Recipe Blend

Date:_____

Name of blend:_____

Size vessel:_____

Carrier oil: _____

Essential oil: _____

Essential oil: _____

Essential oil: _____

Essential oil: _____

Essential oil: _____

Crystal: _____

Other items:_____

Notes about blend:_____

_____

_____

_____

_____

_____

My Own Essential Oil Recipe Blend

Date:_____

Name of blend:_____

Size vessel:_____

Carrier oil: _____

Essential oil: _____

Essential oil: _____

Essential oil: _____

Essential oil: _____

Essential oil: _____

Crystal: _____

Other items:_____

Notes about blend:_____

_____

_____

_____

_____

_____

My Own Essential Oil Recipe Blend

Date: _____

Name of blend: _____

Size vessel: _____

Carrier oil: _____

Essential oil: _____

Essential oil: _____

Essential oil: _____

Essential oil: _____

Essential oil: _____

Crystal: _____

Other items: _____

Notes about blend: _____
_____
_____
_____
_____
_____

My Own Essential Oil Recipe Blend

Date:_____

Name of blend:_____

Size vessel:_____

Carrier oil: _____

Essential oil: _____

Essential oil: _____

Essential oil: _____

Essential oil: _____

Essential oil: _____

Crystal: _____

Other items:_____

Notes about blend:_____

_____

_____

_____

_____

_____

My Own Essential Oil Recipe Blend

Date: _____

Name of blend: _____

Size vessel: _____

Carrier oil: _____

Essential oil: _____

Essential oil: _____

Essential oil: _____

Essential oil: _____

Essential oil: _____

Crystal: _____

Other items: _____

Notes about blend: _____

_____

_____

_____

_____

_____

My Own Essential Oil Recipe Blend

Date:_____

Name of blend:_____

Size vessel:_____

Carrier oil: _____

Essential oil: _____

Essential oil: _____

Essential oil: _____

Essential oil: _____

Essential oil: _____

Crystal: _____

Other items:_____

Notes about blend:_____

_____

_____

_____

_____

_____

My Own Essential Oil Recipe Blend

Date:_____

Name of blend:_____

Size vessel:_____

Carrier oil: _____

Essential oil: _____

Essential oil: _____

Essential oil: _____

Essential oil: _____

Essential oil: _____

Crystal: _____

Other items:_____

Notes about blend:_____

_____

_____

_____

_____

_____

My Own Essential Oil Recipe Blend

Date: _____

Name of blend: _____

Size vessel: _____

Carrier oil: _____

Essential oil: _____

Essential oil: _____

Essential oil: _____

Essential oil: _____

Essential oil: _____

Crystal: _____

Other items: _____

Notes about blend: _____

_____

_____

_____

_____

_____

My Own Essential Oil Recipe Blend

Date:_____

Name of blend:_____

Size vessel:_____

Carrier oil: _____

Essential oil: _____

Essential oil: _____

Essential oil: _____

Essential oil: _____

Essential oil: _____

Crystal: _____

Other items:_____

Notes about blend:_____

_____

_____

_____

_____

_____

My Own Essential Oil Recipe Blend

Date:_____

Name of blend:_____

Size vessel:_____

Carrier oil: _____

Essential oil: _____

Essential oil: _____

Essential oil: _____

Essential oil: _____

Essential oil: _____

Crystal: _____

Other items:_____

Notes about blend:_____

_____

_____

_____

_____

_____

My Own Essential Oil Recipe Blend

Date:_____

Name of blend:_____

Size vessel:_____

Carrier oil: _____

Essential oil: _____

Essential oil: _____

Essential oil: _____

Essential oil: _____

Essential oil: _____

Crystal: _____

Other items:_____

Notes about blend:_____

_____

_____

_____

_____

_____

My Own Essential Oil Recipe Blend

Date:_____

Name of blend:_____

Size vessel:_____

Carrier oil: _____

Essential oil: _____

Essential oil: _____

Essential oil: _____

Essential oil: _____

Essential oil: _____

Crystal: _____

Other items:_____

Notes about blend:_____

_____

_____

_____

_____

_____

My Own Essential Oil Recipe Blend

Date: _____

Name of blend: _____

Size vessel: _____

Carrier oil: _____

Essential oil: _____

Essential oil: _____

Essential oil: _____

Essential oil: _____

Essential oil: _____

Crystal: _____

Other items: _____

Notes about blend: _____
_____
_____
_____
_____
_____

My Own Essential Oil Recipe Blend

Date:_____

Name of blend:_____

Size vessel:_____

Carrier oil: _____

Essential oil: _____

Essential oil: _____

Essential oil: _____

Essential oil: _____

Essential oil: _____

Crystal: _____

Other items:_____

Notes about blend:_____

_____

_____

_____

_____

_____

My Own Essential Oil Recipe Blend

Date:_____

Name of blend:_____

Size vessel:_____

Carrier oil: _____

Essential oil: _____

Essential oil: _____

Essential oil: _____

Essential oil: _____

Essential oil: _____

Crystal: _____

Other items:_____

Notes about blend:_____

_____

_____

_____

_____

_____

My Own Essential Oil Recipe Blend

Date:_____

Name of blend:_____

Size vessel:_____

Carrier oil: _____

Essential oil: _____

Essential oil: _____

Essential oil: _____

Essential oil: _____

Essential oil: _____

Crystal: _____

Other items:_____

Notes about blend:_____

_____

_____

_____

_____

_____

Recommended Suppliers

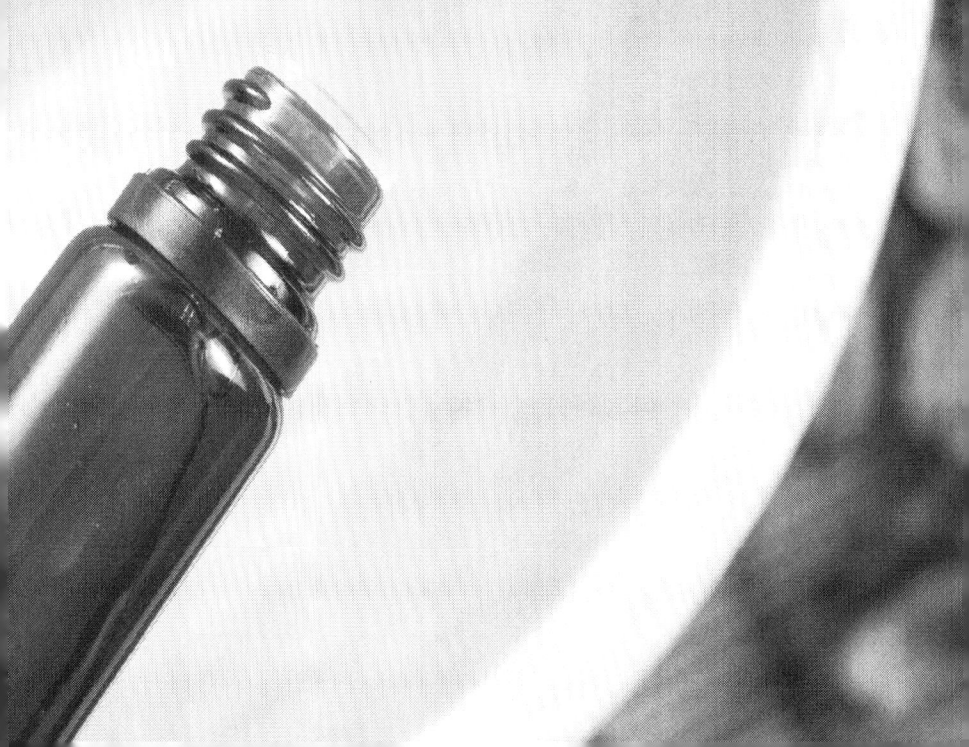

Recommended Suppliers

Here are a few suppliers that I frequent throughout the year while making my blends. I have had lots of success with their products, customer service, as well as great shipping.

Vessels

Hands down Specialty Bottle has been my favorite since I started blending Essential Oils. Their customer service is top notch, there bottles are high quality and the shipping is fast.

Specialty Bottle
http://www.specialtybottle.com/

SKS Bottle & Packaging, Inc.
http://www.sks-bottle.com/

Essential Oils

I cannot stress enough how important it is to purchase high quality, pesticide-free Essential Oils for your blends. These are some of my favorite suppliers.

Pompeii Organics
http://www.pompeiiorganics.com
Owner, Jessica Grill
Importer of high quality, vibrant and organic essential oils. GC/MS reports are available on the website. All products are organic, wildcrafted or unsprayed. Aromatherapy carriers, butters, salts and bottles are also available.

Stillpoint Aromatics
http://www.stillpointaromatics.com/
Co-Owners Joy Mussachio and Cynthia Brownley
Importer of quality, vibrant, organic essential oils. No prepouring. All orders are poured just before shipping. GC/MS reports available on website. All oils are organic, wildcrafted or unsprayed.

Aromatics International
http://www.aromaticsinternational.com/
Owner – Karen Williams
An importer of high quality essential oils. GC/MS reports available on website. All oils are organic, wildcrafted or unsprayed.

Essential Elements Site
http://www.EssentialElementsSite.com
Co-Owners Teresa Miller and Minta Meyer
Here is yet another importer of high quality essential oils. GC/MS reports for all oils are available upon request. Everything they sell is organic, wildcrafted or unsprayed.

Mountain Rose Herbs – Organic Essential Oils
http://www.mountainroseherbs.com/

Aura Cacia
http://www.auracacia.com/

dōTERRA
http://www.doterra.myvoffice.com/mflorapeterson/

CRYSTAL CHIPS

The most frequent question I get is "Where do you get your crystal chips from for the blends?" I usually them from a local store but they can be purchased on Amazon.com as well.

Amazon
http://www.amazon.com/

CARRIER OILS & UNSCENTED LOTIONS

Many of my carrier oils I purchase from Amazon.com. I have found that the shipping is always fast and the qualities of the oils are fantastic.

Amazon
http://www.amazon.com/

EDUCATION

Aromatic Wisdom Institute, School of Creative Aromatherapy
Liz Fulcher, School Director with 22+ years of experience
Email – **Liz@aromaticwisdom.com**
http://www.AromaticWisdomInstitute.com

Aromatherapy Resources

National Association for Holistic Aromatherapy (NAHA)
http://www.naha.org

Alliance of International Aromatherapists (AIA)
http://www.alliance-aromatherapists.org

Aromatherapy Publications

NAHA Aromatherapy Journal
http://www.naha.org

International Journal of Professional Holistic Aromatherapy
http://www.ijpha.com/

Aromatherapy Today
http://www.aromatherapytoday.com

References & Recommended Reading

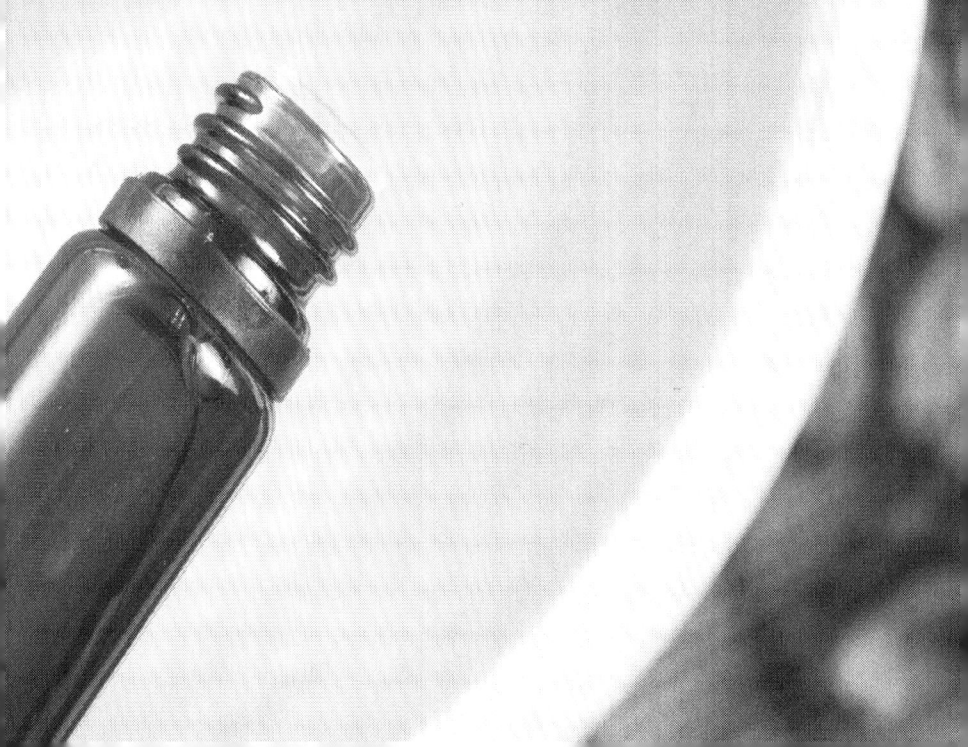

References

Cunningham, Scott. *Incense, Oils and Brews*. Llewellyn Publications, 2002

Fulcher, Liz. Aromatic Wisdom Institute, blog post *Essential Oil Shelf Life*, December 2012.
http://aromaticwisdominstitute.com/essential-oil-self-life

Fulcher, Liz. Aromatic Wisdom Institue, blog post *Blending Guidelines & Dilutions,* August 2012
http://aromaticwisdominstitute.com/blending-guidlines-dilutions

Myer, Sharon. *Essential Oil Blends How to make your own*. http://www.serenearomatherapy.com/essential-oil-blend.html, 2012

Schnaubelt, Kurt. *Advanced Aromatherapy: The Science of Essential Oil Therapy*. Healing Press, 1998

Worwood, Susan & Valerie Ann. *Essential Aromatherapy: A pocket guide to essential oils & aromatherapy*. World Library, 2003

Recommended Reading

Butje, Andrea. Essential Living: Aromatherapy Recipes for Home and Health. Amazon, 2012

Cunningham, Scott. Incense, Oils and Brews. Llewellyn Publications, 2002

Edwards, Victoria H. The Aromatherapy Companion. Story Publishing, 1999

Fulcher, Liz. Aromatic Wisdom Institute Blog, http://www.AromaticWidsomInstitute.com

Moon, Hibiscus. Crystal Grids How and Why They Work. CreateSpace, 2011

Myer, Sharon. Essential Oil Blends How to Make Your Own. http://www.serenearomatherapy.com/essential-oil-blend.html, 2012

Peterson, M. Flora. The Simple Sabbat ~ A Family Friendly Approach to the Eight Pagan Holidays, CreateSpace, 2011

Saches, Allan. The Authoritative Guide to Grapefruit Seed Extract. Life Rhythm, 1997

Schnaubelt, Kurt. Advanced Aromatherapy: The Science of Essential Oil Therapy. Healing Press, 1998

Schnaubelt, Kurt. The Healing Intelligence of Essential Oil. Healing Press, 2011

Wauters, Ambika. The Book of Chakras: Discover the Hidden Forces Within You. Barron's Educational Series, 2002

Worwood, Valerie Ann. Aromatherapy for the Healthy Child. New World Library, 2000

Worwood, Valerie Ann. The Complete Book of Essential Oils and Aromatherapy. New World Library, 1991

Worwood, Susan & Valerie Ann. Essential Aromatherapy: A Pocket Guide to Essential Oils & Aromatherapy. World Library, 2003

The Next Step

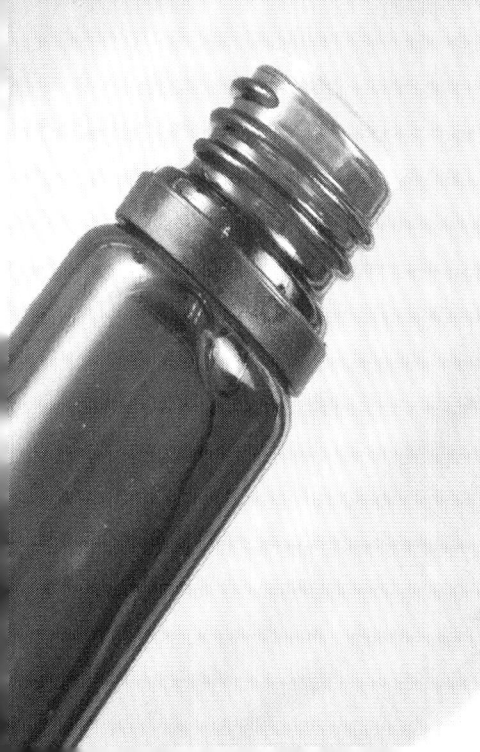

The Next Step

So you have just gotten your feet wet and are itching for more. You want to pursue the enchanted world of Essential Oils.

Here is a good place to start…

The Aromatic Wisdom Institute, School of Creative Aromatherapy in Selinsgrove, PA.
http://www.AromaticWisdomInstitute.com
https://www.Facebook.com/AromaticWisdomInstitute

The Aromatic Wisdom Institute is recognized by the National Association for Holistic Aromatherapy (NAHA) as a qualified school of Aromatherapy and Essential Oil studies.

School Director and Owner, Liz Fulcher strongly emphasizes hand-on experience and encourages her students to tap into personal creativity by developing blends in class. With 22+ years, and counting, of essential oil experience behind her, Liz teaches with warmth, passion and a dedication to her students. She specializes in empowering others to succeed in their own aromatherapy practice.

Currently, classes at the Aromatic Wisdom Institute are in person as well as virtually. Be sure to check the website for all available classes.

Classes:
- 235 Hour Aromatherapy Certification Program
- Therapeutic Uses of Essential Oils
- Energetics of Essential Oils
- Green Cleaning with Essential Oils

Liz publishes a free weekly e-newsletter, A Dose of Aromatic Wisdom, which is bursting with aromatherapy tips, recipes, fragrant affirmations and tools to help boost your aromatherapy practice. To read more or subscribe, please visit:
http://www.AromaticWisdomInstitute.com/newsletter

About Flora

Flora Peterson is an internationally regarded Trainer, Author, Speaker, Spiritual Empowerment Coach and Psychic. Author of numerous books and the founder of the FloraSage Therapies Institute, Flora's dynamic teaching style is highly sought after in the Spiritual Empowerment Coaching & Metaphysical communities.

At the institute Flora teaches Psychic Development courses and personally trains and certifies Spiritual Empowerment Coaches as well as a host of other programs and classes for people from all walks of life. FloraSage Therapies Institute has a strong emphasis in Ethics training for each student, which is a must in this business. A powerful motivational speaker, storyteller and mentor, Flora uses her contagious enthusiasm to empower her clients to live a life that is Fearlessly Inspired.

For a full list of Flora's:
- Private Programs
- Certification Programs
- Classes
- Workshops
- Books
- Meditation CD's
- Affirmation CD's
- Retreats
- Event Calendar
- And much more…

Please visit: https://www.FloraPeterson.com

To Write to the Author

If you wish to contact the author or would like more information about this book, interviews or any other inquiries, please write to the following address:

Flora Peterson
c/o FloraSage Therapies LLC
P.O. Box 2286
Owasso, OK 74055 U.S.A.

http://www.FloraPeterson.com

Flora@FloraPeterson.com

Connect w/ Flora Online

Website

http://www.florapeterson.com

Facebook

https://www.facebook.com/fearlesslyinspired

Twitter

https://twitter.com/PetersonFlora

YouTube

https://www.youtube.com/user/FloraPeterson

The Inner Circle

http://www.mflorapeterson-innercircle.com

The FloraSage Therapies Institute

http://www.florapeterson.com/florasage-therapies-institute/

Made in the USA
Charleston, SC
05 August 2013